Renal Diet
For Beginners

Avoid Kidney Disease with Quick and Tasty Low Sodium, Low Potassium and Low Phosphorous Recipes to Improve Your Kidney Function

Teri Lowe

TABLE OF CONTENTS

INTRODUCTION 6
BREAKFAST 10
    1. Baked Curried Apple Oatmeal Cups 10
    2. Feta Mint Omelette 12
    3. Cherry Berry Bulgur Bowl 13
    4. Sausage Cheese Bake Omelette 15
    5. Italian Breakfast Frittata 16
    6. Mozzarella Cheese Omelette 17
    7. Mexican Scrambled Eggs In Tortilla 18
LUNCH 21
    8. Eggplant Casserole 21
    9. Pizza with Chicken and Pesto 23
    10. Shrimp Quesadilla 25
    11. Grilled Corn on the Cob 27
DINNER 29
    12. Chicken and Broccoli Casserole 29
    13. Pumpkin Bites 31
    14. Feta Bean Salad 32
    15. Sirloin Medallions, Green Squash, and Pineapple 34
MAIN DISHES 37
    16. Spicy Marble Eggs 37
    17. Nutty Oats Pudding 39
    18. Almond Pancakes with Coconut Flakes 40
SNACKS 43

19.	Carrot and Parsnips French Fries	43
20.	Apple & Strawberry Snack	44
21.	Candied Macadamia Nuts	45
22.	Cinnamon Apple Fries	46
23.	Lemon Pops	47

SOUP AND STEW 49

24.	Spicy Chicken Soup	49
25.	Shredded Pork Soup	51
26.	Creamy Chicken Green lettuce Soup	53
27.	Creamy Cauliflower Soup	55

VEGETABLE 57

28.	Curried Cauliflower	57
29.	Chinese Tempeh Stir Fry	59
30.	Egg White Frittata with Penne	60

SIDE DISHES 63

| 31. | Thai-Style Eggplant Dip | 63 |
| 32. | Collard Salad Rolls with Peanut Dipping Sauce | 65 |

SALAD 68

| 33. | Grated carrot salad with Lemon-Dijon vinaigrette | 68 |

FISH & SEAFOOD 71

34.	Fish En' Papillote	71
35.	Tuna Casserole	72
36.	Fish Chili with Lentils	73
37.	Chili Mussels	74
38.	Grilled Cod	75

POULTRY RECIPES 78

| 39. | Lemon Pepper Chicken Legs | 78 |

| 40. | Turkey Broccoli Salad | 80 |
| 41. | Fruity Chicken Salad | 81 |

MEAT RECIPES 82

| 42. | Baked Lamb Chops | 82 |
| 43. | Grilled Lamb Chops with Pineapple | 84 |

BROTHS, CONDIMENT AND SEASONING 87

| 44. | Basil Oil | 87 |
| 45. | Basil Pesto | 89 |

DRINKS AND SMOOTHIES 91

| 46. | Blueberries and Coconut Smoothie | 91 |
| 47. | Creamy Dandelion Greens and Celery Smoothie | 92 |

DESSERT 94

48.	Snickerdoodle chickpea blondies	94
49.	Chocolate chia seed pudding	96
50.	Chocolate-mint truffles	98

INTRODUCTION

Patients with kidney disease should strictly adhere to the guidelines for kidney nutrition. In diabetic kidney nutrition, you learn to control your blood sugar through a healthy diet, especially those that are made for you and your loved ones in need.

You also need to be educated about kidney dietary restrictions so that you are able to avoid foods that contribute too much sodium, potassium and phosphorus to your diet. To learn about kidney disease and its effects on kidney function and health, you need to be aware of the importance of avoiding foods that contain too much sodium, potassium and phosphorus in your diet, as well as the benefits of a healthy diet for your kidneys.

Talk to your kidney dietitian about incorporating the 15 best foods for your kidney nutrition into a healthy eating plan. If you or someone you know is concerned about kidney disease and its impact on kidney function and health, talk to a kidney nutritionist or kidney specialist to find a nutritional plan that works for you.

As a leading board member - a certified kidney specialist - Dr. Gura wants kidney patients to understand the basics of kidney nutrition. If you are diagnosed with kidney disease, adherence to a kidney diet can be a critical part of your treatment. If you suffer from kidney disease or are on kidney dialysis, you must follow a kidney dietary plan.

The diet must be carefully followed, because you can get away with it, but a kidney diet takes into account all aspects of your own health such as blood pressure, cholesterol, blood sugar and blood sugar levels.

People with kidney disease may need to control their diet with certain foods such as fruits, vegetables, whole grains, nuts, beans, legumes and sometimes fluids. Reduce the amount of sodium in your diet and limit your potassium intake, especially in the form of potassium-rich foods.

If you suffer from hyperkalemia due to chronic kidney disease, your doctor may put you on a kidney diet for a short period of time. You may have to go on a kidney dietary plan if you are on dialysis. A low-protein diet is best for people with chronic kidney disease and a high-protein diet is best for dialysis patients, but you need more protein in the form of fruits, vegetables, whole grains, nuts, beans and legumes.

If you consider a whole grain diet, the diet would be fortified with fiber and provide all the fiber needed for its health benefits, and it would possibly provide enough protein without increasing phosphorus content. Diversifying your diet with low sodium and a kidney diet would not only be enriching, but also provide you with everything you need for fiber, for all your health benefits. If you diversify your low-sodium diet and consider whole grains to feed your kidneys, this diet would not only provide enough protein to increase your phosphorus levels, but also provide enough fiber to improve kidney function. A kidney dietary plan for dialysis patients with chronic kidney disease or kidney failure is diversified with low-sodium dietary options.

Remember that patients should include more protein in their diet at the point when dialysis becomes necessary, as this will remove large amounts of protein from the blood. Protein is one of the nutrients that people with kidney disease need to restrict because damaged kidneys cannot remove waste products from protein metabolism. In order to give you the right amount of vitamins and minerals, your dietician may suggest special supplements that are specifically made for you.

As a kidney dietitian, you are often asked which foods are suitable for people with kidney nutrition and what you actually get from these foods. Chefs and dieticians create kidney-friendly meals that are ideal for kidney nutrition. Note that you can easily read the nutritional information on the meals you deliver, as well as the nutritional information for each meal.

If you've come across one of these, take a look at it to create your own kidney-friendly menu. Although kidney nutrition has been used for many years to reduce complications in people with kidney disease, these diets are restrictive and not without criticism.

BREAKFAST

1. Baked Curried Apple Oatmeal Cups

Preparation time: 10 minutes
Cooking time: 20 minutes
Servings: 6

Ingredients
- 3½ cups old-fashioned oats
- 3 tablespoons brown sugar
- 2 teaspoons of your preferred curry powder
- 1/8 teaspoon salt
- 1 cup unsweetened almond milk
- 1 cup unsweetened applesauce
- 1 teaspoon vanilla
- ½ cup chopped walnuts

Directions
1. Preheat the oven to 375°f. Then spray a 12-cup muffin tin with baking spray then set aside.
2. Combine the oats, brown sugar, curry powder, and salt, and mix in a medium bowl.
3. Mix together the milk, applesauce, and vanilla in a small bowl,
4. Stir the liquid ingredients into the dry ingredients and mix until just combined. Stir in the walnuts.

5. Using a scant 1/3 cup for each divide the mixture among the muffin cups.

6. Bake this for 18 to 20 minutes until the oatmeal is firm. Serve.

Nutrition: for 2 oatmeal cups: calories: 296; total fat: 10g; saturated fat: 1g; sodium: 84mg; phosphorus: 236mg; potassium: 289mg; carbohydrates: 45g; fiber: 6g; protein: 8g; sugar: 11g

2. Feta Mint Omelette

Preparation Time: 10 minutes
Cooking Time: 5 minutes
Servings: 1
Ingredients:
- 3 eggs
- 1/4 cup fresh mint, chopped
- 2 tbsp coconut milk
- 1/2 tsp olive oil
- 2 tbsp feta cheese, crumbled
- Pepper
- Salt

Directions:
1. In a bowl, whisk eggs with feta cheese, mint, milk, pepper, and salt.
2. Heat olive oil in a pan over low heat.
3. Pour egg mixture in the pan and cook until eggs are set.
4. Flip omelet and cook for 2 minutes more.
5. Serve and enjoy.

Nutrition: Calories 275 Fat 20 g Carbohydrates 4 g Sugar 2 g Protein 20 g Cholesterol 505 mg phosphorus: 215mg potassium: 269mg sodium: 360mg protein: 19g

3. Cherry Berry Bulgur Bowl

Preparation time: 15 minutes
Cooking time: 15 minutes
Servings: 4

Ingredients
- 1 cup medium-grind bulgur
- 2 cups water
- Pinch salt
- 1 cup halved and pitted cherries or 1 cup canned cherries, drained
- ½ cup raspberries
- ½ cup blackberries
- 1 tablespoon cherry jam
- 2 cups plain whole-milk yogurt

Directions
1. Mix the bulgur, water, and salt in a medium saucepan. Do this in a medium heat. Bring to a boil.
2. Reduce the heat to low and simmer, partially covered, for 12 to 15 minutes or until the bulgur is almost tender. Cover, and let stand for 5 minutes to finish cooking do this after removing the pan from the heat.
3. While the bulgur is cooking, combine the raspberries and blackberries in a medium bowl. Stir the cherry jam into the fruit.

4. When the bulgur is tender, divide among four bowls. Top each bowl with ½ cup of yogurt and an equal amount of the berry mixture and serve.

Nutrition per serving: calories: 242; total fat: 6g; saturated fat: 3g; sodium: 85mg; phosphorus: 237mg; potassium: 438mg; carbohydrates: 44g; fiber: 7g; protein: 9g; sugar: 13g

4. Sausage Cheese Bake Omelette

Preparation Time: 10 minutes
Cooking Time: 45 minutes
Servings: 8
Ingredients:
- 16 eggs
- 2 cups cheddar cheese, shredded
- 1/2 cup salsa
- 1 lb ground sausage
- 1 1/2 cups coconut milk
- Pepper
- Salt

Directions:
1. Preheat the oven to 350 F.
2. Add sausage in a pan and cook until browned. Drain excess fat.
3. In a large bowl, whisk eggs and milk. Stir in cheese, cooked sausage, and salsa.
4. Pour omelet mixture into the baking dish and bake for 45 minutes.
5. Serve and enjoy.

Nutrition: Calories 360 Fat 24 g Carbohydrates 4 g Sugar 3 g Protein 28 g Cholesterol 400 mg phosphorus: 165mg potassium: 370mg sodium: 135mg

5. Italian Breakfast Frittata

Preparation Time: 10 minutes
Cooking Time: 45 minutes
Servings: 4
Ingredients:
- 2 cups egg whites
- 1/2 cup mozzarella cheese, shredded
- 1 cup cottage cheese, crumbled
- 1/4 cup fresh basil, sliced
- 1/2 cup roasted red peppers, sliced
- Pepper
- Salt

Directions:
1. Preheat the oven to 375 F.
2. Add all ingredients into the large bowl and whisk well to combine.
3. Pour frittata mixture into the baking dish and bake for 45 minutes.
4. Slice and serve.

Nutrition: Calories 131 Fat 2 g Carbohydrates 5 g Sugar 2 g Protein 22 g Cholesterol 6 mg phosphorus: 110mg potassium: 117mg sodium: 75mg protein: 7g

6. Mozzarella Cheese Omelette

Preparation Time: 10 minutes
Cooking Time: 5 minutes
Servings: 1

Ingredients:
- 4 eggs, beaten
- 1/4 cup mozzarella cheese, shredded
- 1/4 tsp Italian seasoning
- 1/4 tsp dried oregano
- Pepper
- Salt

Directions:
1. In a small bowl, whisk eggs with salt.
2. Spray pan with cooking spray and heat over medium heat.
3. Pour egg mixture into the pan and cook over medium heat.
4. Once eggs are set then sprinkle oregano and Italian seasoning on top.
5. Cook omelet for 1 minute.
6. Serve and enjoy.

Nutrition: Calories 285 Fat 19 g Carbohydrates 4 g Sugar 3 g Protein 25 g Cholesterol 655 mg Phosphorus: 110mg Potassium: 117mg Sodium: 75mg

7. Mexican Scrambled Eggs In Tortilla

Preparation time: 5 minutes
Cooking time: 2 minutes
Servings: 2

Ingredients

- 2 medium corn tortillas
- 4 egg whites
- 1 teaspoon of cumin
- 3 teaspoons of green chilies, diced
- ½ teaspoon of hot pepper sauce
- 2 tablespoons of salsa
- ½ teaspoon salt

Directions

1. Spray some cooking spray on a medium skillet and heat for a few seconds.
2. Whisk the eggs with the green chilies, hot sauce, and comminute
3. Add the eggs into the pan, and whisk with a spatula to scramble. Add the salt.
4. Cook until fluffy and done (1-2 minutes) over low heat.
5. Open the tortillas and spread 1 tablespoon of salsa on each.
6. Distribute the egg mixture onto the tortillas and wrap gently to make a burrito.
7. Serve warm.

Nutrition: calories: 44.1 kcal carbohydrate: 2.23 g protein: 7.69 g sodium: 854 mg potassium: 189 mg phosphorus: 22 mg dietary fiber: 0.5 g fat: 0.39 g

LUNCH

8. Eggplant Casserole

Preparation Time: 10 minutes
Cooking Time: 25 – 30 minutes
Servings: 4

Ingredients:

- 3 cups of eggplant, peeled and cut into large chunks
- 2 egg whites
- 1 large egg, whole
- ½ cup of unsweetened vegetable
- ¼ tsp of sage
- ½ cup of breadcrumbs
- 1 tbsp. of margarine, melted
- 1/4 tsp garlic salt

Directions:

1. Preheat the oven at 350F/180C.
2. Place the eggplants chunks in a medium pan, cover with a bit of water and cook with the lid covered until tender. Drain from the water and mash with a tool or fork.
3. Beat the eggs with the non-dairy vegetable cream, sage, salt, and pepper. Whisk in the eggplant mush.
4. Combine the melted margarine with the breadcrumbs.

5. Bake in the oven for 20-25 minutes or until the casserole has a golden-brown crust.

Nutrition: Calories: 186 Carbohydrate: 19 g Protein: 7 g Fat: 9 g Sodium: 503 mg Potassium: 230 mg Phosphorus: 62 mg

9. Pizza with Chicken and Pesto

Preparation Time: 10 minutes
Cooking Time: 25 minutes
Servings: 4

Ingredients:
- 1 ready-made frozen pizza dough
- 2/3 cup cooked chicken, chopped
- 1/2 cup of mango bell pepper, diced
- 1/2 cup of green bell pepper, diced
- 1/4 cup of purple onion, chopped
- 2 tbsp. of green basil pesto
- 1 tbsp. of chives, chopped
- 1/3 cup of parmesan or Romano cheese, grated
- 1/4 cup of mozzarella cheese
- 1 tbsp. of olive oil

Directions:
1. Thaw the pizza dough according to instructions on the package.
2. Heat the olive oil in a pan and sauté the peppers and onions for a couple of minutes. Set aside
3. Once the pizza dough has thawed, spread the Bali pesto over its surface.
4. Top with half of the cheese, the peppers, the onions, and the chicken. Finish with the rest of the cheese.
5. Bake at 350F/180C for approx. 20 minutes (or until crust and cheese are baked).

6. Slice in triangles with a pizza cutter or sharp knife and serve.

Nutrition: Calories: 225 Carbohydrate: 13.9 g Protein: 11.1 g Fat: 12 g Sodium: 321 mg Potassium: 174 mg Phosphorus: 172 mg

10. Shrimp Quesadilla

Preparation Time: 10 minutes
Cooking Time: 10 minutes
Servings: 2

Ingredients:

- 5 oz. of shrimp, shelled and deveined
- 4 tbsp. of Mexican salsa
- 2 tbsp. of fresh cilantro, chopped
- 1 tbsp. of lemon juice
- 1 tsp of ground cumin
- 1 tsp of cayenne pepper
- 2 tbsp. of unsweetened soy yogurt or creamy tofu
- 2 medium corn flour tortillas
- 2 tbsp. of low-fat cheddar cheese

Directions:

1. Mix the cilantro, cumin, lemon juice, and cayenne in a Ziploc bag to make your marinade.

2. Put the shrimps and marinate for 10 minutes.

3. Heat a pan over medium heat with some olive oil and toss in the shrimp with the marinade. Let cook for a couple of minutes or as soon as shrimps have turned pink and opaque.

4. Add the soy cream or soft tofu to the pan and mix well. Remove from the heat and keep the marinade aside.

5. Heat tortillas in the grill or microwave for a few seconds.

6. Place 2 tbsp. of salsa on each tortilla. Top one tortilla with the shrimp mixture and add the cheese on top.

7. Stack one tortilla against each other (with the spread salsa layer facing the shrimp mixture).

8. Transfer this on a baking tray and cook for 7-8 minutes at 350F/180C to melt the cheese and crisp up the tortillas.

9. Serve warm.

Nutrition: Calories: 255 Carbohydrate: 21 g Fat: 9 g Protein: 24 g Sodium: 562 g Potassium: 235 mg Phosphorus: 189 mg

11. Grilled Corn on the Cob

Preparation Time: 5 minutes
Cooking Time: 20 minutes
Servings: 4

Ingredients:
- 4 frozen corn on the cob, cut in half
- ½ tsp of thyme
- 1 tbsp. of grated parmesan cheese
- ¼ tsp of black pepper

Directions:
1. Combine the oil, cheese, thyme, and black pepper in a bowl.
2. Place the corn in the cheese/oil mix and roll to coat evenly.
3. Fold all 4 pieces in aluminum foil, leaving a small open surface on top.
4. Place the wrapped corns over the grill and let cook for 20 minutes.
5. Serve hot.

Nutrition: Calories: 125 Carbohydrate: 29.5 g Protein: 2 g Fat: 1.3 g Sodium: 26 g Potassium: 145 mg Phosphorus: 91.5 mg

DINNER

12. Chicken and Broccoli Casserole

Preparation Time: 15 minutes
Cooking Time: 45 minutes – 1 hour
Servings: 1

Ingredients:
- 2 cups of rice (cooked)
- 3 chicken breasts
- 2 cups of broccoli
- 1 onion (diced)
- 2 eggs
- 2 cups of cheddar cheese
- 2 tbsp of butter
- 1-2 tbsp of parmesan cheese

Directions:
1. Heat the oven to 350 degrees-Fahrenheit
2. Add the broccoli to a bowl and cover it with plastic wrap. Microwave the broccoli for 2-3 minutes.
3. Dice the onion and add it with the chicken and the butter in the pa.
4. Cook the chicken for 15 minutes.
5. Once the chicken is cooked, mix it, broccoli, and rice together, and add to a greased casserole dish.

6. Add the grated cheese into the casserole dish and stir well.

7. Add the parmesan cheese on top.

8. Place the casserole dish in the oven for 30-45 minutes.

Nutrition: Calories: 349 Fat: 12g Carbs: 14g Protein: 44g Sodium: 980mg Potassium: 713mg Phosphorus: 451mg

13. Pumpkin Bites

Preparation Time: 10 minutes
Cooking Time: 5 minutes
Servings: 12

Ingredients:

- 8 oz cream cheese
- 1 tsp vanilla
- 1 tsp pumpkin pie spice
- 1/4 cup coconut flour
- 1/4 cup erythritol
- 1/2 cup pumpkin puree
- 4 oz butter

Directions:

1. Add all ingredients into the mixing bowl and beat using hand mixer until well combined.
2. Scoop mixture into the silicone ice cube tray and place it in the refrigerator until set.
3. Serve and enjoy.

Nutrition: Calories 149 Fat 14.6 g Carbohydrates 8.1 gSugar 5.4 g Protein 2 g Cholesterol 41 mg Phosphorus: 66mg Potassium: 77mg Sodium: 55mg

14. Feta Bean Salad

Preparation Time: 5 minutes
Cooking Time: 20 minutes
Servings: 2

Ingredients:

- 1 tbsp of olive oil
- 2 egg whites (boiled)
- 1 cup of green beans (8 oz)
- 1 tbsp of onion
- 1/2 red chili
- 1/8 cup of cilantro
- 1 1/2 tbsp lime juice
- 1/4 tbsp of black pepper

Directions:

1. Remove the ends off the green beans and cut them into small pieces.
2. Chop the onion, cilantro, and chili and mix it.
3. Use a steamer to cook green beans for 5- 10 minutes and rinse with cold water once done.
4. Place all the mixed dry ingredients together in two serving bowls.
5. Chop the egg whites up and place them on top of the salad with crumbled feta.
6. Drizzle a pinch of olive oil with black pepper on top.

Nutrition: Calories: 255 Fat: 24g Carbs: 8g Protein: 5g Sodium: 215.6mg Potassium: 211mg Phosphorus: 125mg

15. Sirloin Medallions, Green Squash, and Pineapple

Preparation Time: 10 minutes

Cooking Time: 40 minutes

Servings: 4

Ingredients:

- 1 lb. of sirloin medallions
- 1 medium baby marrows
- 1 yellow squash
- ½ onion
- 8 oz of thinly sliced pineapple
- 3 tbsp of olive oil
- 2 tsp of ginger
- ½ tsp of salt
- 1 garlic clove

Directions:

1. Retrieve thinly sliced pineapple rings from a can and drain. Set the juice aside.
2. Slice garlic and ginger into fine pieces.
3. Mix the pineapple juice, ginger, garlic, salt, and olive oil together in a bowl to create a dressing for the sirloin medallions.
4. Add the sirloin medallions to the marinade and let it sit for 10-15 minutes.

5. Heat the oven to 450 degrees-Fahrenheit and line 2 oven trays with parchment paper.
6. Chop the squash into little ½-inch circles and place it on the parchment paper—drizzle 1tbsp of olive oil on top of it.
7. Cut the onion into small wedges, add to the tray and drizzle with olive oil.
8. Add pineapple rings next to the squash on the first tray and roast for 6 minutes.
9. Remove the pan and turn the squash and pineapple over. Add the onion onto the tray and roast it for another 5 minutes. Close the fruit and vegetables with foil to lock in the heat and set aside.
10. Remove sirloin medallions from the marinade. Line another oven tray pan with parchment paper and place the sirloin medallions on top.
11. Cook for 5 minutes and flip the sirloin to cook for another 5 minutes on the other side.
12. Serve the sirloin medallions with the vegetables and pineapple on a platter.

Nutrition: Calories: 264 Fat: 12g Carbs: 14g Protein: 25g Sodium: 150mg Potassium: 685mg Phosphorus: 257mg

MAIN DISHES

16. Spicy Marble Eggs

Preparation Time: 15 minutes
Cooking Time: 2 hours
Servings: 12

Ingredients:

- 6 medium-boiled eggs, unpeeled, cooled
- For the Marinade
- 2 oolong black tea bags
- 3 Tbsp. brown sugar
- 1 thumb-sized fresh ginger, unpeeled, crushed
- 3 dried star anise, whole
- 2 dried bay leaves
- 3 Tbsp. light soy sauce
- 4 Tbsp. dark soy sauce
- 4 cups of water
- 1 dried cinnamon stick, whole
- 1 tsp. salt
- 1 tsp. dried Szechuan peppercorns

Directions:

1. Using the back of a metal spoon, crack eggshells in places to create a spider web effect. Do not peel. Set aside until needed.
2. Pour marinade into large Dutch oven set over high heat. Put lid partially on. Bring water to a rolling boil, about 5 minutes. Turn off heat.

3. Secure lid. Steep ingredients for 10 minutes.
4. Using a slotted spoon, fish out and discard solids. Cool marinade completely to room proceeding.
5. Place eggs into an airtight non-reactive container just small enough to snugly fit all these in.
6. Pour in marinade. Eggs should be completely submerged in liquid. Discard leftover marinade, if any. Line container rim with generous layers of saran wrap. Secure container lid.
7. Chill eggs for 24 hours before using.
8. Extract eggs and drain each piece well before using, but keep the rest submerged in the marinade.

Nutrition: Calories: 75 kcal Protein: 4.05 g Fat: 4.36 g Carbohydrates: 4.83 g

17. Nutty Oats Pudding

Preparation Time: 5 minutes
Cooking Time: 0 minutes
Servings: 3 -5

Ingredients:

- ¼ cup rolled oats
- 1 tablespoon yogurt, fat-free
- 1 ½ tablespoon natural peanut butter
- ¼ cup dry almond milk
- 1 teaspoon peanuts, finely chopped
- ½ cup of water

Directions:

1. Using a microwaveable-safe bowl, put together peanut butter and dry almond milk. Whisk well. Add in water to achieve a smooth consistency. Add in oats.
2. Cover bowl with plastic wrap. Create a small hole for the steam to escape.
3. Place inside the microwave oven for 1 minute on high powder.
4. Continue heating, this time on medium power for 90 seconds. Let sit for 5 minutes.
5. To serve, spoon an equal amount of cereals in a bowl top with peanuts and yogurt.

Nutrition: Calories: 70 kcal Protein: 4.25 g Fat: 3.83 g Carbohydrates: 6.78 g

18. Almond Pancakes with Coconut Flakes

Preparation: Time: 5 minutes

Cooking Time: 10 minutes

Servings: 6

Ingredients:

- 1 overripe banana, mashed
- 2 eggs, yolks, and whites separated
- ½ cup unsweetened applesauce
- 1 cup almond flour, finely milled
- ¼ cup of water
- ¼ tsp. coconut oil
- Garnish
- 2 Tbsp. blanched almond flakes
- Dash of cinnamon powder
- ¼ cup coconut flakes, sweetened
- Pinch of sea salt
- Pure maple syrup, use sparingly

Directions:

1. Whisk egg whites until soft peaks form.
2. Except for egg whites and coconut oil, combine remaining ingredients in another bowl. Mix until batter comes together.
3. Gently fold in egg whites. Make sure that you don't over mix, or the pancake will become dense and chewy.

4. Pour oil into a nonstick skillet set over medium heat.
5. Wait for the oil to heat up before dropping in approximately ½ cup of batter. Cook until each side are set, and bubbles form in the center. Turn on the other side then cook for another 2 minutes.
6. Transfer flapjacks to a plate. Repeat step until all batter is cooked. Pour in more oil into the skillet only if needed. This recipe should yield between 4 to 6 medium-sized pancakes.
7. Stack pancakes. Pour the desired amount of pure maple syrup on top. Garnish each stack with cinnamon-flavored almond-coconut flakes just before serving.
8. For the garnish, set the oven to 350°F for at least 10 minutes before use. Line a baking sheet with parchment paper. Set aside.
9. Mix almond and coconut flakes together in a bowl. Spread mixture evenly on a prepared baking sheet.
10. Bake for 7 to 10 minutes until flakes turn golden brown. Stir almond and coconut flakes once midway through roasting to prevent over-browning.
11. Remove the baking sheet from the oven. Cool almond and coconut flakes for at least 10 minutes before sprinkling in cinnamon powder and salt. Toss to combine. Set aside.

Nutrition: Calories: 62 kcal Protein: 2.24 g Fat: 4.01 g

SNACKS

19. Carrot and Parsnips French Fries

Preparation Time: 15 minutes
Cooking Time: 20 minutes
Servings: 2

Ingredients:
- 6 large carrots
- 6 large parsnips
- 2 tablespoons extra virgin olive oil
- ½ teaspoon of sea salt

Directions:
1. Chop the carrots and parsnips into 2-inch slices and then cut each into thin sticks.
2. Toss together the carrots and parsnip sticks with extra virgin olive oil and salt in a bowl and spread into a baking sheet lined with parchment paper.
3. Bake the sticks at 425° for about 20 minutes or until browned.

Nutrition: Calories: 179 Fat: 4g Carbs: 14g Protein: 11g Sodium: 27.3mg Potassium: 625mg Phosphorus: 116mg

20. Apple & Strawberry Snack

Preparation Time: 5 minutes
Cooking Time: 2 minutes
Servings: 1

Ingredients:

- ½ apple, cored and sliced
- 2-3 strawberries
- dash of ground cinnamon
- 2-3 drops stevia 2-3 drops

Directions:

1. In a bowl, mix strawberries and apples and sprinkle with stevia and cinnamon.
2. Microwave for about 1-2 minutes. Serve warm.

Nutrition: Calories: 145 Fat: 0.8 g Carbs: 34.2 g Protein: 1.6 g Sodium: 20 mg Potassium: 0mg Phosphorus: 0mg

21. Candied Macadamia Nuts

Preparation Time: 5 minutes
Cooking Time: 15 minutes
Servings: 2

Ingredients:
- 2 cups macadamia nuts
- 1 tablespoon extra-virgin olive oil
- 2 tablespoons honey

Directions:
1. Toss ingredients in bowl and spread into a baking dish.
2. Bake for 15 minutes at 350°F.
3. Let cool before serving.

Nutrition: Calories: 200 Fat: 18 Carbs: 10g Protein: 1g Sodium: 5 mg Potassium: 55mg Phosphorus: 10mg

22. Cinnamon Apple Fries

Preparation Time: 5 minutes
Cooking Time: 15 minutes
Servings: 1

Ingredients:
- 1 apple, sliced thinly
- Dash of cinnamon
- Stevia

Directions:
1. Coat apple slices with cinnamon and stevia.
2. Bake for 15 minutes or until tender and crispy at 325 degrees F.

Nutrition: Calories: 146 Fat: 0.7 g Carbs: 36.4 g Protein: 1.6 g Sodium: 10 mg Potassium: 100mg Phosphorus: 0mg

23. Lemon Pops

Preparation Time: 5 minutes
Cooking Time: 5 minutes
Servings: 1

Ingredients:
- 4 tablespoons fresh lemon juice
- Powdered stevia

Directions:
1. Mix mango or lemon juice and stevia and pour into molds.
2. Freeze until firm.

Nutrition: Calories: 46 Fat: 0.2g Carbs: 16g Protein: 0.9g Sodium: 3.7mg Potassium: 104mg Phosphorus: 11mg

SOUP AND STEW

24. Spicy Chicken Soup

Preparation Time: 10 minutes
Cooking Time: 5 minutes
Servings: 4

Ingredients:

- 2 cups cooked chicken, shredded
- 1/2 cup half and half
- 4 cups chicken broth
- 1/3 cup hot sauce
- 3 tbsp. butter
- 4 oz. cream cheese
- Pepper
- Salt

Directions:

1. Add half and half, broth, hot sauce, butter, and cream cheese into the blender and blend until smooth.
2. Pour blended mixture into the saucepan and cook over medium heat until just hot.
3. Add chicken stir well. Season soup with pepper and salt.
4. Serve and enjoy.

Nutrition: Calories 361 Fat 25.6 g Carbohydrates 3.3 g Sugar 1.1 g Protein 28.4 g Cholesterol 119 mg Phosphorus: 110mg Potassium: 117mg Sodium: 75mg

25. Shredded Pork Soup

Preparation Time: 10 minutes
Cooking Time: 8 hours
Servings: 8
Ingredients:
- 1 lb. pork loin
- 8 cups chicken broth
- 2 tsp fresh lime juice
- 1 1/2 tsp garlic powder
- 1 1/2 tsp onion powder
- 1 1/2 tsp chili powder
- 1 1/2 tsp cumin
- 1 jalapeno pepper, minced
- 1 cup onion, chopped
- 3 Red bell peppers, chopped

Directions:
1. Add Red bell peppers, jalapeno, and onion into the slow cooker and stir well.
2. Place meat on top of the tomato mixture.
3. Pour remaining ingredients on top of the meat.
4. Cover slow cooker and cook on low for 8 hours.
5. Remove meat from slow cooker and shred using a fork.
6. Return shredded meat to the slow cooker and stir well.

7. Serve and enjoy.

Nutrition: Calories 199 Fat 9.6 g Carbohydrates 6.3 g Sugar 3.1 g Protein 21.2 g Cholesterol 45 mg Phosphorus: 140mg Potassium: 127mg Sodium: 95mg

26. Creamy Chicken Green lettuce Soup

Preparation Time: 10 minutes
Cooking Time: 10 minutes
Servings: 6

Ingredients:
- 3 cups cooked chicken, shredded
- 1/8 tsp nutmeg
- 4 cup chicken broth
- 1/2 cup parmesan cheese, shredded
- 8 oz. cream cheese
- 1/4 cup butter
- 4 cup baby green lettuce, chopped
- 1 tsp garlic, minced
- Pepper
- Salt

Directions:
1. Melt butter in a saucepan over medium heat.
2. Add green lettuce and garlic and cook until green lettuce is wilted.
3. Add parmesan cheese and cream cheese and stir until cheese is melted.
4. Add remaining ingredients and stir everything well and cook for 5 minutes.
5. Season soup with pepper and salt.
6. Serve and enjoy.

Nutrition: Calories 361 Fat 25.6 g Carbohydrates 2.8 g Sugar 0.6 g Protein 29.5 g Cholesterol 121 mg Phosphorus: 110mg Potassium: 117mg Sodium: 75mg

27. Creamy Cauliflower Soup

Preparation Time: 10 minutes
Cooking Time: 4 hours
Servings: 5

Ingredients:

- 6 cups cauliflower florets
- 4 oz. mascarpone cheese
- 1 1/2 cup cheddar cheese, shredded
- 1/4 tsp mustard powder
- 3 cups of water
- 1 tsp garlic, minced
- Pepper
- Salt

Directions:

1. Add cauliflower, mustard powder, water, and garlic into the slow cooker and stir well.
2. Cover and cook on low for 4 hours.
3. Stir in cheddar cheese and mascarpone cheese.
4. Puree the soup using an immersion blender until smooth.
5. Season soup with pepper and salt.
6. Serve and enjoy.

Nutrition: Calories 208 Fat 14.3 g Carbohydrates 7.7 g Sugar 3.1 g Protein 13.5 g Cholesterol 47 mg Phosphorus: 210mg Potassium: 157mg Sodium: 85mg

VEGETABLE

28. Curried Cauliflower

Preparation time: 5 minutes
Cooking time: 20 minutes
Servings: 4 servings

Ingredients:

- 1 tsp. turmeric
- 1 diced onion
- 1 tbsp. chopped fresh cilantro
- 1 tsp. cumin
- ½ diced chili
- ½ cup water
- 1 minced garlic clove
- 1 tbsp. coconut oil
- 1 tsp. garam masala
- 2 cups cauliflower florets

Directions:

1. Add the oil to a skillet on medium heat.
2. Sauté the onion and garlic for 5 minutes until soft.
3. Add the cumin, turmeric and garam masala and stir to release the aromas.
4. Now add the chili to the pan along with the cauliflower.

5. Stir to coat.

6. Pour in the water and reduce the heat to a simmer for 15 minutes.

7. Garnish with cilantro to serve.

Nutrition: Calories: 108 kcal; Total Fat: 7 g; Saturated Fat: 0 g; Cholesterol: 0 mg; Sodium: 35 mg; Total Carbs: 11 g; Fiber: 0 g; Sugar: 0 g; Protein: 2 g

29. Chinese Tempeh Stir Fry

Preparation time: 5 minutes
Cooking time: 15 minutes
Servings: 2 servings
Ingredients:

- 2 oz. sliced tempeh
- 1 cup cooked rice
- 1 minced garlic clove
- ½ cup green onions
- 1 tsp. minced fresh ginger
- 1 tbsp. coconut oil
- ½ cup corn

Directions:

1. Heat the oil in a skillet or wok on a high heat and add the garlic and ginger.
2. Sauté for 1 minute.
3. Now add the tempeh and cook for 5-6 minutes before adding the corn for a further 10 minutes.
4. Now add the green onions and serve over rice.

Nutrition: Calories: 304 kcal; Total Fat: 4 g; Saturated Fat: 0 g; Cholesterol: 0 mg; Sodium: 91 mg; Total Carbs: 35 g; Fiber: 0 g; Sugar: 0 g; Protein: 10 g

30. Egg White Frittata with Penne

Preparation time: 15 minutes
Cooking time: 30 minutes
Servings: 4 servings

Ingredients:

- Egg whites- 6
- Rice almond milk – ¼ cup
- Chopped fresh parsley – 1 tbsp.
- Chopped fresh thyme – 1 tsp
- Chopped fresh chives – 1 tsp
- Ground black pepper
- Olive oil – 2 tsp.
- Small sweet onion – ¼, chopped
- Minced garlic – 1 tsp
- Boiled and chopped red bell pepper – ½ cup
- Cooked penne – 2 cups

Directions:

1. Preheat the oven to 350f.
2. In a bowl, whisk together the egg whites, rice almond milk, parsley, thyme, chives, and pepper.
3. Heat the oil in a skillet.
4. Sauté the onion, garlic, red pepper for 4 minutes or until they are softened.
5. Add the cooked penne to the skillet.

6. Pour the egg mixture over the pasta and shake the pan to coat the pasta.

7. Leave the skillet on the heat for 1 minute to set the frittata's bottom and then transfer the skillet to the oven.

8. Bake the frittata for 25 minutes, or until it is set and golden brown.

9. Serve.

Nutrition: Calories: 170 kcal; Total Fat: 3 g; Saturated Fat: 0 g; Cholesterol: 0 mg; Sodium: 90 mg; Total Carbs: 25 g; Fiber: 0 g; Sugar: 0 g; Protein: 10 g

SIDE DISHES

31. Thai-Style Eggplant Dip

Preparation Time: 10 minutes
Cooking Time: 30 minutes
Servings: 4

Ingredients:
- 1 pound Thai eggplant (or Japanese or Chinese eggplant)
- 2 tablespoons rice vinegar
- 2 teaspoons sugar
- 1 teaspoon low-sodium soy sauce
- 1 jalapeño pepper
- 2 garlic cloves
- ¼ cup chopped basil
- Cut vegetables for serving

Directions:
1. Preheat the oven to 475°F
2. Pierce the eggplant in several places with a skewer or knife. Place on a rimmed baking sheet and cook until soft, about 30 minutes.
3. Let cool, cut in half, and scoop out the flesh of the eggplant into a blender.
4. Add the rice vinegar, sugar, soy sauce, jalapeño, garlic, and basil to the blender. Process until smooth. Serve with cut vegetables

5. Lower sodium tip: If you need to lower your sodium further, omit the soy sauce to lower the sodium to 3mg.

Nutrition: Calories: 40; Total Fat: 0g; Saturated Fat: 0g; Cholesterol: 0mg; Carbohydrates: 10g; Fiber: 4g; Protein: 2g; Phosphorus: 34mg; Potassium: 284mg; Sodium: 47mg

32. Collard Salad Rolls with Peanut Dipping Sauce

Preparation Time: 10 minutes
Cooking Time: 10 minutes
Servings: 4

Ingredients:
- FOR THE DIPPING SAUCE
- ¼ cup peanut butter
- 2 tablespoons honey
- Juice of 1 lime
- ¼ teaspoon red chili flakes
- FOR THE SALAD ROLLS
- 4 ounces' extra-firm tofu
- 1 bunch collard greens
- 1 cup thinly sliced purple cabbage
- 1 cup bean sprouts
- 2 carrots, cut into matchsticks
- ½ cup cilantro leaves and stems

Directions:
1. TO MAKE THE DIPPING SAUCE
2. In a blender, combine the peanut butter, honey, lime juice, chili flakes, and process until smooth. Put 1 to 2 tablespoons of water as desired for consistency.
3. TO MAKE THE SALAD ROLLS
4. Using paper towels, press the excess moisture from the tofu. Cut into ½-inch-thick matchsticks.
5. Remove any tough stems from the collard greens and set aside.

6. Arrange all of the ingredients within reach. Cup one collard green leaf in your hand, and add a couple pieces of the tofu and a small amount each of the cabbage, bean sprouts, and carrots. Top with a couple cilantro sprigs, and roll into a cylinder. Place each roll, seam-side down, on a serving platter while you assemble the rest of the rolls. Serve with the dipping sauce.
7. Substitution tip: To lower the potassium, omit the cabbage and use only 1 carrot, which will drop the potassium to 208mg.

Nutrition: Calories: 174; Total Fat: 9g; Saturated Fat: 2g; Cholesterol: 0mg; Carbohydrates: 20g; Fiber: 5g; Protein: 8g; Phosphorus: 56mg; Potassium: 284mg; Sodium: 42mg

SALAD

33. Grated carrot salad with Lemon-Dijon vinaigrette

Preparation time: 15 minutes

Cooking time: 10 minutes

Servings: 8 servings

Ingredients:

- 9 small carrots (14 cm), peeled
- 2 tbsp. 1/2 teaspoon Dijon mustard
- 1 C. lemon juice
- 2 tbsp. extra virgin olive oil
- 1-2 tsp. honey (to taste)
- ¼ tsp. salt
- ¼ tsp. freshly ground pepper (to taste)
- 2 tbsp. chopped parsley
- 1 green onion, thinly sliced

Directions:

1. Grate the carrots in a food processor.

2. In a salad bowl, mix Dijon mustard, lemon juice, honey, olive oil, salt, and pepper. Add the carrots, fresh parsley, and green onions. Stir to coat well. Cover and refrigerate until ready to be serve.

Nutrition: Energy: 61 g, Proteins: 1 g, Carbohydrates: 7 g, fibbers: 1 g, Total Fat: 4 g, Sodium: 88 mg, Phosphorus: 22 mg, Potassium: 197 mg

FISH & SEAFOOD

34. Fish En' Papillote

Preparation Time: 15 minutes
Cooking Time: 20 minutes
Servings: 3

Ingredients:

- 10 oz. snapper fillet
- 1 tablespoon fresh dill, chopped
- 1 white onion, peeled, sliced
- ½ teaspoon tarragon
- 1 tablespoon olive oil
- 1 teaspoon salt
- ½ teaspoon hot pepper
- 2 tablespoons sour cream

Directions:

1. Make the medium size packets from parchment and arrange them in the baking tray. Cut the snapper fillet into 3 and sprinkle them with salt, tarragon, and hot pepper.
2. Put the fish fillets in the parchment packets. Then top the fish with olive oil, sour cream, sliced onion, and fresh dill. Bake the fish for 20 minutes at 355F. Serve.

Nutrition: Calories 204 Fat 8.2g Carbs 4.6g Protein 27.2g Phosphorus 138.8 mg Potassium 181.9 mg Sodium 59.6 mg

35. Tuna Casserole

Preparation Time: 15 minutes

Cooking Time: 35 minutes

Servings: 4

Ingredients:
- ½ cup Cheddar cheese, shredded
- 2 Red bell peppers, chopped
- 7 oz. tuna filet, chopped
- 1 teaspoon ground coriander
- ½ teaspoon salt
- 1 teaspoon olive oil
- ½ teaspoon dried oregano

Directions:
1. Brush the casserole mold with olive oil. Mix up together chopped tuna fillet with dried oregano and ground coriander.
2. Place the fish in the mold and flatten well to get the layer. Then add chopped Red bell peppers and shredded cheese. Cover the casserole with foil and secure the edges. Bake the meal for 35 minutes at 355F. Serve.

Nutrition: Calories 260 Fat 21.5g Carbs 2.7g Protein 14.6g Phosphorus 153 mg Potassium 311 mg   Sodium 600 mg

36. Fish Chili with Lentils

Preparation Time: 10 minutes
Cooking Time: 30 minutes
Servings: 4

Ingredients:
- 1 red pepper, chopped
- 1 yellow onion, diced
- 1 teaspoon ground black pepper
- 1 teaspoon butter
- 1 jalapeno pepper, chopped
- ½ cup lentils
- 3 cups chicken stock
- 1 teaspoon salt
- 1 tablespoon tomato paste
- 1 teaspoon chili pepper
- 3 tablespoons fresh cilantro, chopped
- 8 oz. cod, chopped

Directions:
1. Place butter, red pepper, onion, and ground black pepper in the saucepan. Roast the vegetables for 5 minutes over medium heat.
2. Then add chopped jalapeno pepper, lentils, and chili pepper. Mix up the mixture well and add chicken stock and tomato paste. Stir until homogenous. Add cod. Close the lid and cook chili for 20 minutes over medium heat.

Nutrition: Calories 187 Fat 2.3g Carbs 21.3g Protein 20.6g Phosphorus 50 mg Potassium 281 mg Sodium 43.8 mg

37. Chili Mussels

Preparation Time: 7 minutes
Cooking Time: 10 minutes
Servings: 4

Ingredients:

- 1-pound mussels
- 1 chili pepper, chopped
- 1 cup chicken stock
- ½ cup almond milk
- 1 teaspoon olive oil
- 1 teaspoon minced garlic
- 1 teaspoon ground coriander
- ½ teaspoon salt
- 1 cup fresh parsley, chopped
- 4 tablespoons lemon juice

Directions:

1. Pour almond milk into the saucepan. Add chili pepper, chicken stock, olive oil, minced garlic, ground coriander, salt, and lemon juice.
2. Bring the liquid to boil and add mussels. Boil the mussel for 4 minutes or until they will open shells. Then add chopped parsley and mix up the meal well. Remove it from the heat.

Nutrition: Calories 136 Fat 4.7g Fiber 0.6g Carbs 7.5gProtein 15.3g Phosphorus 180.8 mg Potassium 312.5 mg Sodium 319.6 mg

38. Grilled Cod

Preparation Time: 10 min
Cooking Time: 10 minutes
Servings: 4

Ingredients:

- 2 (8 ounce) fillets cod, cut in half
- 1 tablespoon oregano
- ½ teaspoon lemon pepper
- ¼ teaspoon ground black pepper
- 2 tablespoons olive oil
- 1 lemon, juiced
- 2 tablespoons chopped green onion (white part only)

Directions:

1. Season both sides of cod with oregano, lemon pepper, and black pepper. Set fish aside on a plate. Heat butter in a small saucepan over medium heat, stir in lemon juice and green onion, and cook until onion is softened, about 3 minutes.

2. Place cod onto oiled grates and grill until fish is browned and flakes easily, about 3 minutes per side; baste with olive oil mixture frequently while grilling. Allow cod to rest off the heat for about 5 minutes before serving.

Nutrition: Calories 92, Total Fat 7.4g, Saturated Fat 1g, Cholesterol 14mg, Sodium 19mg, Total Carbohydrate 2.5g,

Dietary Fiber 1g, Total Sugars 0.5g, Protein 5.4g, Calcium 25mg, Iron 1mg, Potassium 50mg, Phosphorus 36 mg

POULTRY RECIPES

39. Lemon Pepper Chicken Legs

Preparation Time: 5 minutes
Cooking Time: 25 minutes
Servings: 4

Ingredients:
- ½ tsp. garlic powder
- 2 tsp. baking powder
- 8 chicken legs
- 4 tbsp. salted butter, melted
- 1 tbsp. lemon pepper seasoning

Directions:
1. In a small container add the garlic powder and baking powder, then use this mixture to coat the chicken legs. Lay the chicken in the basket of your fryer.
2. Cook the chicken legs at 375°F for twenty-five minutes. Halfway through, turn them over and allow to cook on the other side.
3. When the chicken has turned golden brown, test with a thermometer to ensure it has reached an ideal temperature of 165°F. Remove from the fryer.
4. Mix together the melted butter and lemon pepper seasoning and toss with the chicken legs until the chicken is coated all over. Serve hot.

Nutrition: Calories: 132 Fat: 16 g Carbs: 20 g Protein: 48 g Calcium 79mg, Phosphorous 132mg, Potassium 127mg   Sodium: 121 mg

40. Turkey Broccoli Salad

Preparation Time: 10 minutes
Cooking Time: 00 minutes
Servings: 4

Ingredients:

- 8 cups broccoli florets
- 3 cooked skinless, boneless chicken breast halves, cubed
- 6 green onions, chopped
- 1 cup mayonnaise
- ¼ cup apple cider vinegar
- ¼ cup honey

Directions:

1. Combine broccoli, chicken and green onions in a large bowl.
2. Whisk mayonnaise, vinegar, and honey together in a bowl until well blended.
3. Pour mayonnaise dressing over broccoli mixture; toss to coat.
4. Cover and refrigerate until chilled, if desired. Serve

Nutrition: Calories 133, Sodium 23mg, Dietary Fiber 1.6g, Total Sugars 7.7g, Protein 6.2g, Calcium 24mg, Potassium 157mg Phosphorus 148 mg

41. Fruity Chicken Salad

Preparation Time: 10 minutes
Cooking Time: 5 minutes
Servings: 3

Ingredients:

- 4 skinless, boneless chicken breast halves - cooked and diced
- 1 stalk celery, diced
- 4 green onions, chopped
- 1 Golden Delicious apple - peeled, cored and diced
- 1/3 cup seedless green grapes, halved
- 1/8 teaspoon ground black pepper
- 3/4 cup light mayonnaise

Directions:

1. In a large container, add the celery, chicken, onion, apple, grapes, pepper, and mayonnaise.
2. Mix all together. Serve!

Nutrition: Calories 196, Sodium 181mg, Total Carbohydrate 15.6g, Dietary Fiber 1.2g, Total Sugars 9.1g, Protein 13.2g, Calcium 13mg, Iron 1mg, Potassium 115mg, Phosphorus 88 mg

MEAT RECIPES

42. Baked Lamb Chops

Preparation time: 10 min
Cooking Time: 45 minutes
Servings: 4

Ingredients:

- 2 eggs
- 2 teaspoons Worcestershire sauce
- 8 (5.5 ounces) lamb chops
- 2 cups graham crackers

Directions:

1. Preheat oven to 375 degrees F.
2. In a medium bowl, combine the eggs and the Worcestershire sauce; stir well. Dip each lamb chop in the sauce and then lightly dredge in the graham crackers. Then arrange them in a 9x13-inch baking dish.
3. Bake at 375 degrees F for 20 minutes, turn chops over and cook for 20 more minutes, or to the desired doneness.

Nutrition: Calories176, Total Fat 5.7g, Saturated Fat 1.4g, Cholesterol 72mg, Sodium 223mg, Total Carbohydrate 21.9g, Dietary Fiber 0.8g, Total Sugars 9.2g, Protein 9.1g, Vitamin D

5mcg, Calcium 17mg, Iron 2mg, Potassium 121mg, Phosphorus 85 mg

43. Grilled Lamb Chops with Pineapple

Preparation time: 15 min

Cooking Time: 55 minutes

Servings: 4

Ingredients:

- 1 lemon, zest and juiced
- 2 tablespoons chopped fresh oregano
- 2 cloves garlic, minced
- salt and black pepper to taste
- 8 (3 ounces) lamb chops
- 1/2 cup fresh unsweetened pineapple juice
- 1 cup pineapples

Directions:

1. Whisk together the lemon zest and juice, oregano, garlic, salt, and black pepper in a bowl; pour into a resealable plastic bag. Add the lamb chops, coat with the marinade, squeeze out excess air, and seal the bag.

2. Set aside to marinate.

3. Preheat an outdoor grill for medium-high heat, and lightly oil the grate.

4. Bring the pineapple juice in a small saucepan over high heat.

5. Reduce heat to medium-low, and continue simmering until the liquid has reduced to half of its original volume, about 45 minutes.

6. Stir in the pineapples and set aside.

7. Remove the lamb from the marinade and shake off excess.

8. Discard the remaining marinade.

9. Cook the chops on the preheated grill until they start to firm and are reddish-pink and juicy in the center, about 4 minutes per side for medium rare.

10. Serve the chops drizzled with the pineapple reduction.

Nutrition: Calories 69, Total Fat 1.6g, Saturated Fat 0.5g, Cholesterol 17mg, Sodium 16mg, Total Carbohydrate 8.5g, Dietary Fiber 1.4g, Total Sugars 5.1g, Protein 5.9g, Calcium 37mg, Iron 1mg, Potassium 163mg, Phosphorus 65 mg

BROTHS, CONDIMENT AND SEASONING

44. Basil Oil

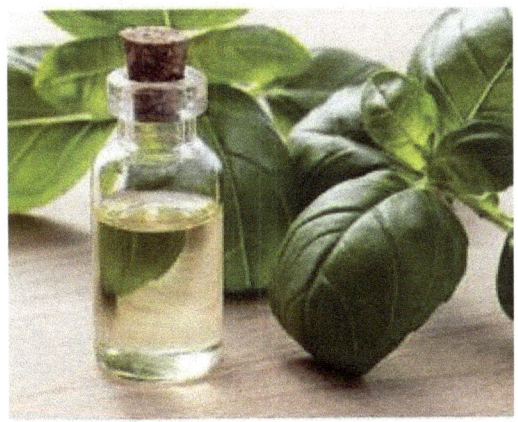

Preparation Time: 15 minutes
Cooking Time: 4 minutes
Servings: 3

Ingredients:
- 2 cups olive oil
- 2½ cups fresh basil leaves patted dry

Directions:
1. Put the olive oil plus basil leaves in a food processor or blender, and pulse until the leaves are coarsely chopped.
2. Transfer these to a medium saucepan, and place over medium heat. Heat the oil, occasionally stirring, until it

just starts to simmer along the edges, about 4 minutes. Remove, then let it stand until cool, about 2 hours.
3. Pour the oil through a fine-mesh sieve or doubled piece of cheesecloth into a container. Store the basil oil in an airtight glass container in the refrigerator for up to 2 months.
4. Before using for dressings, remove the oil from the refrigerator and let it come to room temperature, or for cooking, scoop out cold spoonsful.

Nutrition: Calories: 40Fat: 5gSodium: 0gCarbohydrates: 0g Phosphorus: 0g Potassium: 0g Protein: 0g

45. Basil Pesto

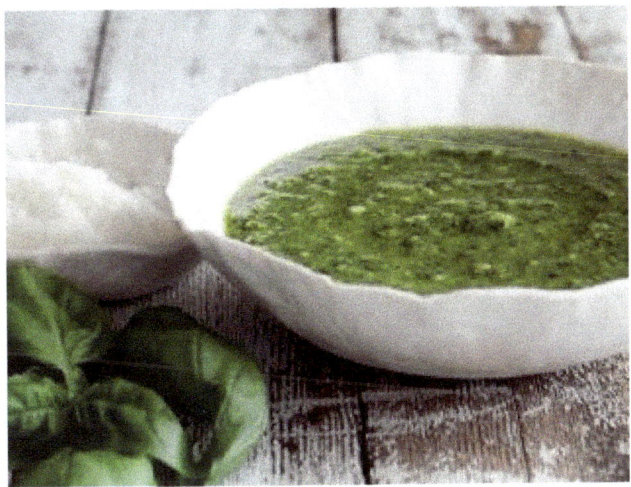

Preparation Time: 15 minutes

Cooking Time: 0 minutes

Servings: 1 ½ cups

Ingredients:

- 2 cups gently packed fresh basil leaves
- 2 garlic cloves
- 2 tablespoons pine nuts
- ¼ cup olive oil
- 2 tablespoons freshly squeezed lemon juice

Directions:

1. Pulse the basil, garlic, plus pine nuts using a food processor or blender within about 3 minutes. Drizzle the olive oil into this batter, and pulse until thick paste forms.
2. Put the lemon juice, and pulse until well blended. Store the pesto in a sealed glass container in the refrigerator for up to 2 weeks.

Nutrition: Calories: 22 Fat: 2g Sodium: 0mg Carbohydrates: 0g Phosphorus: 3mg Potassium: 10mg Protein: 0g

DRINKS AND SMOOTHIES

46. Blueberries and Coconut Smoothie

Preparation Time: 5 minutes

Cooking Time: 3 minutes

Servings: 5

Ingredients:

- 1 cup of frozen blueberries, unsweetened
- 1 cup stevia or erythritol sweetener
- 2 cups coconut almond milk (canned)
- 1 cup of fresh green lettuce leaves
- 2 tablespoon shredded coconut (unsweetened)
- 3/4 cup water

Directions:

1. Place all ingredients from the list in food-processor or in your strong blender.
2. Blend for 45 - 60 seconds or to taste.
3. Ready for drink! Serve!

Nutrition: Calories: 190, Carbohydrates: 8g, Proteins: 3g, Fat: 18g, Fiber: 2g, Calcium 79mg, Phosphorous 216mg, Potassium 207mg Sodium: 121 mg

47. Creamy Dandelion Greens and Celery Smoothie

Preparation Time: 10 minutes

Cooking Time: 3 minutes

Servings: 2

Ingredients:

- 1 handful of raw dandelion greens
- 2 celery sticks
- 2 tablespoon chia seeds
- 1 small piece of ginger, minced
- 1/2 cup almond milk
- 1/2 cup of water
- 1/2 cup plain yogurt

Directions:

1. Rinse and clean dandelion leaves from any dirt; add in a high-speed blender.
2. Clean the ginger; keep only inner part and cut in small slices; add in a blender.
3. Blend all remaining ingredients until smooth.
4. Serve and enjoy!

Nutrition: Calories: 58, Carbohydrates: 5g, Proteins: 3g, Fat: 6g, Fiber: 3gCalcium 29mg, Phosphorous 76mg, Potassium 27mg Sodium: 121 mg

DESSERT

48. Snickerdoodle chickpea blondies

Servings: 15

Preparation time: 10 minutes

Cooking time: 30 to 35 minutes

Ingredients:

- 1 (15-ounce) can chickpeas, drained and rinsed
- 3 tablespoons nut butter of choice
- ¾ teaspoon baking powder
- 2 teaspoons vanilla extract
- 1/8 teaspoon baking soda
- ¾ cup brown sugar
- 1 tablespoon unsweetened applesauce
- 1/4 cup ground flaxseed meal
- 21/4 teaspoons cinnamon

Directions:

1. Preheat the oven to 350°f. Grease an 8-by-8-inch baking pan.

2. Blend all ingredients in a food processor until very smooth. Scoop into the prepared baking pan.

3. Bake until the tops are medium golden brown, 30 to 35 minutes. Allow the brownies to cool completely before cutting.

Nutrition: calories: 85; total fat 2g; saturated fat: 0g; cholesterol: 0mg; sodium: 7mg; potassium: 62mg; total carbohydrate: 16g; fiber: 2g; protein: 3g

49. Chocolate chia seed pudding

Preparation time: 15 minutes, plus 3 to 5 hours or overnight to rest

Cooking time: 0 minutes

Servings: 4

Ingredients:

- 1 1/2 cups unsweetened vanilla almond milk
- 1/4 cup unsweetened cocoa powder
- 1/4 cup maple syrup (or substitute any sweetener)
- 1/2 teaspoon vanilla extract
- 1/3 cup chia seeds
- 1/2 cup strawberries
- 1/4 cup blueberries
- 1/4 cup raspberries
- 2 tablespoons unsweetened coconut flakes
- 1/4 to 1/2 teaspoon ground cinnamon (optional)

Directions:

1. Add the almond milk, cocoa powder, maple syrup, and vanilla extract to a blender and blend until smooth. Whisk in chia seeds.

2. In a small bowl, gently mash the strawberries with a fork. Distribute the strawberry mash evenly to the bottom of 4 glass jars.

3. Pour equal portions of the blended almond milk-cocoa mixture into each of the jars and let the pudding rest in the refrigerator until it achieves a pudding like consistency, at least 3 to 5 hours and up to overnight.

Nutrition: calories: 189; total fat 7g; saturated fat: 2g; cholesterol: 0mg; sodium: 60mg; potassium: 232mg; total carbohydrate: 28g; fiber: 10g; protein: 6g

50. Chocolate-mint truffles

Preparation time: 45 minutes
Cooking time: 5 hours
Servings: 60 small truffles

Ingredients:

- 14 ounces semisweet chocolate, coarsely chopped
- ¾ cup half-and-half
- 1/2 teaspoon pure vanilla extract
- 1 1/2 teaspoon peppermint extract
- 2 tablespoons unsalted butter, softened
- ¾ cup naturally unsweetened or dutch-process cocoa powder

Directions:

1. Place semisweet chocolate in a large heatproof bowl.

2. Microwave in four 15-second increments, stirring after each, for a total of 60 seconds. Stir until almost completely melted. Set aside.

3. In a small saucepan over medium heat, heat the half-and-half, whisking occasionally, until it just begins to boil. Remove from the heat, then whisk in the vanilla and peppermint extracts.

4. Pour the mixture over the chocolate and, using a wooden spoon, gently stir in one direction.

5. Once the chocolate and cream are smooth, stir in the butter until it is combined and melted.

6. Cover with plastic wrap pressed on the top of the mixture, and then let it sit at room temperature for 30 minutes.

7. After 30 minutes, place the mixture in the refrigerator until it is thick and can hold a ball shape, about 5 hours.

8. Line a large baking sheet with parchment paper or a use a silicone baking mat. Set aside.

9. Remove the mixture from the refrigerator. Place the cocoa powder in a bowl.

10. Scoop 1 teaspoon of the ganache and, using your hands, roll into a ball. Roll the ball in the cocoa powder, the place on the prepared baking sheet. (you can coat your palms with a little cocoa powder to prevent sticking).

11. Serve immediately or cover and store at room temperature for up to 1 week.

Nutrition: calories: 21; total fat 2g; saturated fat: 1g; cholesterol: 2mg; sodium: 2mg; potassium: 21mg; total carbohydrate: 2g; fiber: 1g; protein: 0g

Lightning Source UK Ltd.
Milton Keynes UK
UKHW020813150321
380363UK00001B/15